BODY DISCIPLINE

WHAT DOES THE BIBLE SAY ABOUT EXERCISE & FITNESS?

BY TOREMA THOMPSON

BODY DISCIPLINE: WHAT DOES THE BIBLE SAY ABOUT EXERCISE & FITNESS?

ISBN: 978-1-8384368-1-0

First published in the UK by Pura Track Publishing in April 2021.

This book is intended for educational purposes only. Individuals reading this book are solely responsible for their own decisions & actions.

For business enquiries, email: questions@toremathompson.uk

WWW.TOREMATHOMPSON.UK

"I discipline my body like an athlete, training it to do what it should. Otherwise, I fear that after preaching to others I myself might be disqualified."

(1 Corinthians 9:27, NLT)

FIRST THINGS FIRST...

You are a spirit.

You have a soul.

You live in a body.

> "Now may the God of peace make you holy in every way, and may your whole spirit and soul and body be kept blameless until our Lord Jesus Christ comes again." (1 Thessalonians 5:23, NLT)

You are a three-part being made in God's image.

God desires that all three be preserved until the Lord comes again.

God desires all three to be used for His glory.

YOU ARE A SPIRIT.

Your spirit man is who you are.

As a child of God, saved by grace through faith, this is the part of you that has become completely new.

> *Therefore if any man be in Christ, he is a new creature: old things are passed away; behold, all things are become new. (2 Corinthians 5:17)*

When Christ saved you, His Spirit joined with yours making you no longer just a human being, but a supernatural being—God's very own.

> *So you have not received a spirit that makes you fearful slaves. Instead, you received God's Spirit when he adopted you as his own children. Now we call him, "Abba, Father." For his Spirit joins with our spirit to affirm that we are God's children. (Romans 8:15-16)*

YOU HAVE
A SOUL.

Simply put, your soul is:

- Your mind.
- Your will.
- Your emotions.

Your soul did not automatically change when you were saved. It is in the *process* of transformation.

> And be not conformed to this world: but be ye transformed by the renewing of your mind, that ye may prove what is that good, and acceptable, and perfect, will of God. (Romans 12:2).

The soul is the domain of *choice*. If you choose to allow your spirit to dictate, you will see prosperity in your body.

> Beloved, I pray that you may prosper in every way and [that your body] may keep well, even as [I know] your soul keeps well and prospers. (3 John 1:2, AMPC)

YOU LIVE
IN A BODY.

Your physical body is your earthly house. It is the vehicle through which you carry out your God given assignment. If your car stops working how will you get from A to B? If your body becomes sick and weak, how will you be able to do all that God has ordained for you to do on the earth?

> **For we know that if the tent which is our earthly home is destroyed (dissolved), we have from God a building, a house not made with hands, eternal in the heavens. (2 Corinthians 5:1, AMPC)**

As well as being your earthly home, your body is also the temple of the Holy Ghost. In fact, it is no longer your body but HIS.

> **What? know ye not that your body is the temple of the Holy Ghost which is in you, which ye have of God, and ye are not your own? For ye are bought with a price: therefore glorify God in your body, and in your spirit, which are God's. (1 Corinthians 6:19-20)**

YOU WILL GIVE AN ACCOUNT.

Your body does not belong to you because Christ paid for it with His own blood. As with anything else the Lord gives, you must have the mentality that you are simply a STEWARD.

> *So then every one of us shall give account of himself to God. (Romans 14:12)*

> *Moreover, it is [essentially] required of stewards that a man should be found faithful [proving himself worthy of trust]. (1 Corinthians 4:2, AMPC)*

> *God will destroy anyone who destroys this temple. For God's temple is holy, and you are that temple. (1 Corinthians 3:17, NLT)*

PAUSE AND REFLECT.

The Lord has given you personal stewardship over your body.

Take a few moments now to think about your stewardship over your body...

Have you been a good steward? Have you been faithful with that which He has given to you?

- Do you feed your body what it needs?
- Do you give it the rest that it requires?
- Do you give it the amount of physical activity that it needs?
- Do you clean and care for it the way it needs?

If not, take this time to repent if necessary.

Decide that, from today, you will not only see your body as something the Lord has given you stewardship over, but that you will also make a conscious effort to be a <u>faithful</u> steward of your body.

Ask the Lord: *What do I need to change to be a better steward of my body?*

"Physical training is good, but training for godliness is much better, promising benefits in this life and in the life to come."

(1 Timothy 4:8, NLT)

Physical training is good.

Bodily exercise has some value.

When compared to training for godliness, physical training takes a back seat...

Nevertheless, **body discipline** *is* still beneficial.

As a believer, you are never to place more emphasis on the physical than the spiritual, but the Bible is clear that there are benefits to engaging in physical activity and exercise.

Training yourself physically improves your physical fitness. Physical fitness relates to your ability to perform daily tasks effectively and without undue fatigue, enabling you to do that which God has called you to do.

> *She girds herself with strength [spiritual, mental, and physical fitness for her God-given task] and makes her arms strong and firm. (Proverbs 31:17, AMPC)*

GOD CAN
HELP YOU.

- Do you struggle with **body discipline**?
- Do you dislike working out?
- Maybe you want to work out but find yourself too busy?
- Or perhaps you are on the other extreme where you are addicted to training?

The good news is, wherever you fall on the scale above, the Lord CAN help you find that healthy balance. All He needs from you is your willingness, and He'll do the rest (if you let Him).

> *And so, dear brothers and sisters, I plead with you to give your bodies to God because of all he has done for you. Let them be a living and holy sacrifice—the kind he will find acceptable. This is truly the way to worship him. (Romans 12:1, NLT)*

> *For I can do everything through Christ, who gives me strength. (Philippians 4:13, NLT)*

"No discipline is enjoyable
while it is happening—it's
painful! But afterward there
will be a peaceful harvest of
right living for those who are
trained in this way."

(Hebrews 12:11, NLT)

As with spiritual discipline, physical discipline also requires time and dedication.

You may not reach all your goals at once, but you will see the results if you don't quit!

> *So let's not get tired of doing what is good. At just the right time we will reap a harvest of blessing if we don't give up. (Galatians 6:9, NLT)*

Try to keep an eternal perspective in your journey with **body discipline**. Remember that, ultimately, looking after your earth suit will enable you to be more available for the work of the Kingdom!

> *And whatever you do [no matter what it is] in word or deed, do everything in the name of the Lord Jesus and in [dependence upon] His Person, giving praise to God the Father through Him. (Colossians 3:17, AMPC)*

About the Author

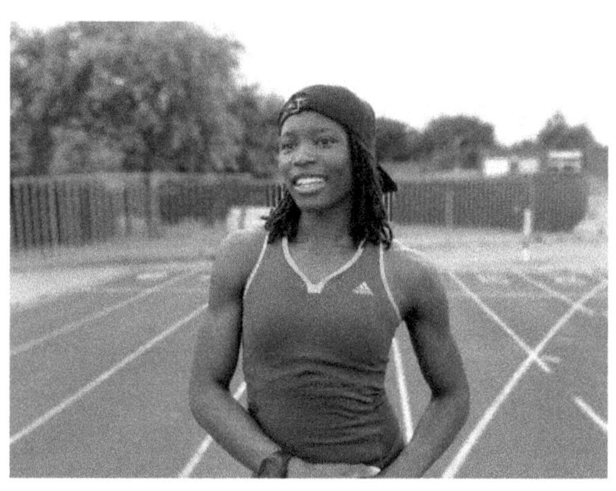

L3 Personal Trainer | L2 Fitness Instructor |
UKA L2 Athletics Coach Speed

Torema Thompson is an athlete, author, adviser, coach, and entrepreneur.

Through her personal brand, she helps athletes and fitness enthusiasts to go from newbies to masters in their athletics and fitness.

Through her teaching ministry, Pura*T International, she equips God's people with the Word of Truth.

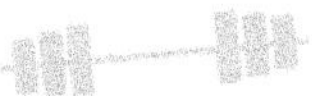

CONNECT WITH TOREMA ONLINE:

"@ToremaThompson"

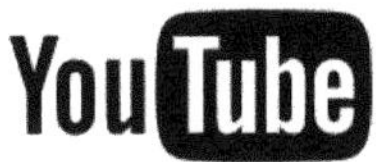

TRAIN WITH TOREMA:

www.toremathompson.uk/coaching

GET YOUR FREE PDF VERSION OF THIS BOOK!

https://www.toremathompson.uk/bodydiscipline

PURA*T INTERNATIONAL:

https://www.puratinternational.org.uk/

FAITH & FITNESS VIDEO SERIES:

www.ingramcontent.com/pod-product-compliance
Ingram Content Group UK Ltd.
Pitfield, Milton Keynes, MK11 3LW, UK
UKHW021036270726
13967UKWH00013B/2661

9 781838 436810